The Definitive Me
Meat Recipe

Healthy and Tasty Meat Recipes 1
Diet

Raymond Morton

Table of contents

Cocoa Lamb

Prep time: 10 minutes I **Cooking time:** 35 minutes I **Servings:** 4

Ingredients:

- ½ cup veggie stock
- 1 pound lamb stew meat, cubed
- 1 cup radishes, cubed
- 1 tablespoon cocoa powder
- Black pepper to the taste
- 1 yellow onion, chopped
- 1 tablespoon olive oil
- 2 garlic cloves, minced
- 1 tablespoon parsley, chopped

Directions:

1. Heat up a pan with the oil over medium-high heat, add the onion and the garlic, toss and sauté for 5 minutes.
2. Add the meat, toss and brown for 2 minutes on each side.
3. Add the stock and the other ingredients, toss, bring to a simmer and cook over medium heat for 25 minutes more.
4. Divide everything between plates and serve.

Nutrition info per serving: calories 340, fat 12.4, fiber 9.3, carbs 33.14, protein 20

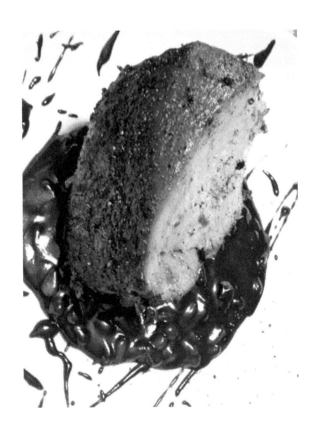

Lemon Pork with Jalapeno Artichokes

Prep time: 10 minutes I **Cooking time:** 25 minutes I **Servings:** 4

Ingredients:

- 2 pounds pork stew meat, cut into strips
- 2 tablespoons avocado oil
- 1 tablespoon lemon juice
- 1 tablespoon lemon zest, grated
- 1 cup artichokes, cut into quarters
- 1 red onion, chopped
- 2 garlic cloves, minced
- ½ teaspoon chili powder
- Black pepper to the taste
- 1 teaspoon sweet paprika
- 1 jalapeno, chopped
- ¼ cup veggie stock
- ¼ cup rosemary, chopped

Directions:

1. Heat up a pan with the oil over medium-high heat, add the onion and the garlic, toss and sauté for 4 minutes.
2. Add the meat, artichokes, chili powder, the jalapeno and the paprika, toss and cook for 6 minutes more.
3. Add the rest of the ingredients, toss, bring to a simmer and cook over medium heat for 15 minutes more.
4. Divide the whole mix into bowls and serve.

Nutrition info per serving: calories 350, fat 12, fiber 4.3, carbs 35.7, protein 14.5

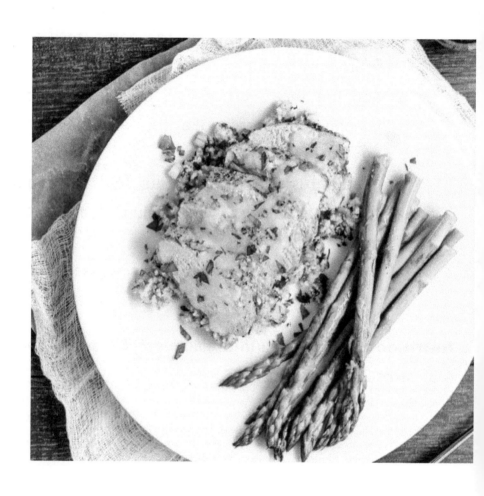

Pork with Cilantro Sauce

Prep time: 10 minutes I **Cooking time:** 20 minutes I
Servings: 4

Ingredients:

- 2 pounds pork stew meat, roughly cubed
- 1 cup cilantro leaves
- 4 tablespoons olive oil
- 1 tablespoon pine nuts
- 1 tablespoon parmesan, grated
- 1 tablespoon lemon juice
- 1 teaspoon chili powder
- Black pepper to the taste

Directions:

1. In a blender, combine the cilantro with the pine nuts, 3 tablespoons oil, parmesan and lemon juice and pulse well.
2. Heat up a pan with the remaining oil over medium heat, add the meat, chili powder and the black pepper, toss and brown for 5 minutes.
3. Add the cilantro sauce, and cook over medium heat for 15 minutes more, stirring from time to time.
4. Divide the pork between plates and serve right away.

Nutrition info per serving: calories 270, fat 6.6, fiber 7, carbs 12.6, protein 22.4

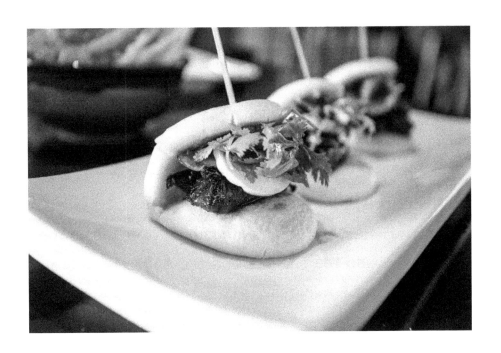

Pork with Mango Mix

Prep time: 10 minutes I **Cooking time:** 25 minutes I **Servings:** 4

Ingredients:

- 2 shallots, chopped
- 2 tablespoons avocado oil
- 1 pound pork stew meat, cubed
- 1 mango, peeled and roughly cubed
- 2 garlic cloves, minced
- 1 cup tomatoes, and chopped
- Black pepper to the taste
- ½ cup basil, chopped

Directions:

1. Heat up a pan with the oil over medium heat, add the shallots and the garlic, toss and cook for 5 minutes.
2. Add the meat, toss and cook for 5 minutes more.
3. Add the rest of the ingredients, toss, bring to a simmer and cook over medium heat for 15 minutes more.
4. Divide the mix into bowls and serve.

Nutrition info per serving: calories 361, fat 11, fiber 5.1, carbs 16.8, protein 22

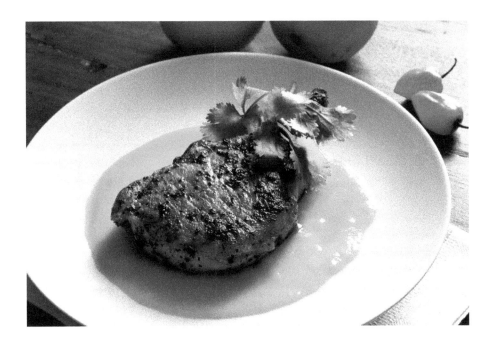

Rosemary Pork

Prep time: 10 minutes I **Cooking time:** 35 minutes I **Servings:** 4

Ingredients:

- 1 red onion, cut into wedges
- 2 sweet potatoes, peeled and cut into wedges
- 4 pork chops
- 1 tablespoon rosemary, chopped
- 1 tablespoon lemon juice
- 2 teaspoons olive oil
- Black pepper to the taste
- 2 teaspoons thyme, chopped
- ½ cup veggie stock

Directions:

1. In a roasting pan, combine the pork chops with the potatoes, onion and the other ingredients and toss gently.
2. Bake at 400 degrees F for 35 minutes, divide everything between plates and serve.

Nutrition info per serving: calories 410, fat 14.7, fiber 14.2, carbs 15.3, protein 33.4

Pork with Chickpeas

Prep time: 10 minutes I **Cooking time:** 25 minutes I
Servings: 4

Ingredients:

- 1 pound pork stew meat, cubed
- 1 cup chickpeas, cooked
- 1 yellow onion, chopped
- 1 tablespoon olive oil
- Black pepper to the taste
- 10 ounces tomatoes, chopped
- 2 tablespoons cilantro, chopped

Directions:

1. Heat up a pan with the oil over medium-high heat, add the onion, toss and sauté for 5 minutes.
2. Add the meat, toss and cook for 5 minutes more.
3. Add the rest of the ingredients, toss, simmer over medium heat for 15 minutes, divide everything into bowls and serve.

Nutrition info per serving: calories 476, fat 17.6, fiber 10.2, carbs 35.7, protein 43.8

Lamb and Kale

Prep time: 10 minutes I **Cooking time:** 35 minutes I

Servings: 4

Ingredients:

- 1 cup kale, torn
- 1 pound lamb chops
- ½ cup veggie stock
- 2 tablespoons tomato passata
- 1 yellow onion, sliced
- 1 tablespoon olive oil
- A pinch of black pepper

Directions:

1. Grease a roasting pan with the oil, arrange the lamb chops inside, also add the kale and the other ingredients and toss gently.
2. Bake everything at 390 degrees F for 35 minutes, divide between plates and serve.

Nutrition info per serving: calories 275, fat 11.8, fiber 1.4, carbs 7.3, protein 33.6

Chili Lamb

Prep time: 10 minutes I **Cooking time:** 45 minutes I **Servings:** 4

Ingredients:

- 2 pounds lamb stew meat, cubed
- 1 tablespoon avocado oil
- 1 teaspoon chili powder
- 1 teaspoon hot paprika
- 2 red onions, roughly chopped
- 1 cup veggie stock
- ½ cup tomato passata
- 1 tablespoon cilantro, chopped

Directions:

1. Heat up a pot with the oil over medium heat, add the onion and the meat and brown for 10 minutes.
2. Add the chili powder and the other ingredients except the cilantro, toss, bring to a simmer and cook over medium heat for 35 minutes more.
3. Divide the mix into bowls and serve with the cilantro sprinkled on top.

Nutrition info per serving: calories 463, fat 17.3, fiber 2.3, carbs 8.4, protein 65.1

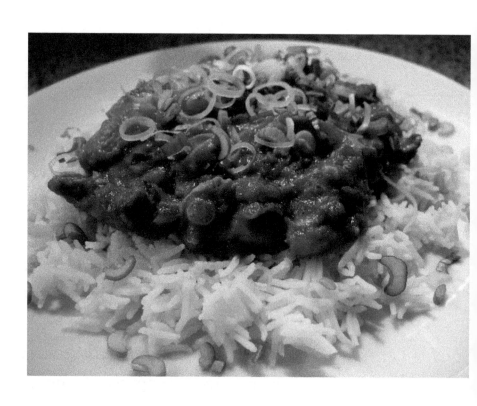

Pork and Leeks

Prep time: 10 minutes I **Cooking time:** 45 minutes I
Servings: 4

Ingredients:

- 2 pounds pork stew meat, roughly cubed
- 2 leeks, sliced
- 2 tablespoons olive oil
- 2 garlic cloves, minced
- 1 teaspoon sweet paprika
- 1 tablespoon parsley, chopped
- 1 cup veggie stock
- Black pepper to the taste

Directions:

1. Heat up a pan with the oil over medium heat, add the leeks, garlic and the paprika, toss and cook for 10 minutes.
2. Add the meat and brown it for 5 minutes more.
3. Add the remaining ingredients, toss, simmer over medium heat for 30 minutes, divide everything into bowls and serve.

Nutrition info per serving: calories 577, fat 29.1, fiber 1.3, carbs 8.2, protein 67.5

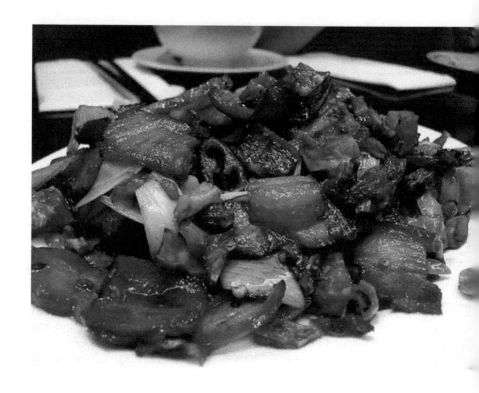

Pork and Peas

Prep time: 10 minutes I **Cooking time:** 25 minutes I
Servings: 4

Ingredients:

- 4 pork chops
- 2 tablespoons olive oil
- 2 shallots, chopped
- 1 cup snow peas
- 1 cup veggie stock
- 2 tablespoons tomato paste
- 1 tablespoon parsley, chopped

Directions:

1. Heat up a pan with the oil over medium heat, add the shallots, toss and sauté for 5 minutes.
2. Add the pork chops and brown for 2 minutes on each side.
3. Add the rest of the ingredients, bring to a simmer and cook over medium heat for 15 minutes.
4. Divide the mix between plates and serve.

Nutrition info per serving: calories 357, fat 27, fiber 1.9, carbs 7.7, protein 20.7

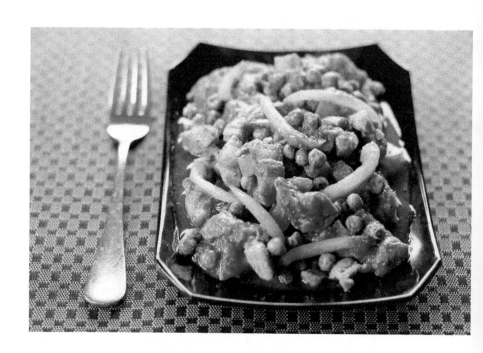

Pork and Corn

Ingredients:

- 4 pork chops
- 1 cup veggie stock
- 1 cup corn
- 1 tablespoon mint, chopped
- 1 teaspoons sweet paprika
- Black pepper to the taste
- 1 tablespoon olive oil

Directions:

1. Put the pork chops in a roasting pan, add the rest of the ingredients, toss, introduce in the oven and bake at 380 degrees F for 1 hour.
2. Divide everything between plates and serve.

Nutrition info per serving: calories 356, fat 14, fiber 5.4, carbs 11.0, protein 1

Dill Lime Lamb

Prep time: 10 minutes I **Cooking time:** 25 minutes I **Servings:** 4

Ingredients:

- Juice of 2 limes
- 1 tablespoon lime zest, grated
- 1 tablespoon dill, chopped
- 2 garlic cloves, minced
- 2 tablespoons olive oil
- 2 pounds lamb meat, cubed
- 1 cup cilantro, chopped
- Black pepper to the taste

Directions:

1. Heat up a pan with the oil over medium-high heat, add the garlic and the meat and brown for 4 minutes on each side.
2. Add the lime juice and the other ingredients and cook for 15 minutes more stirring often.
3. Divide everything between plates and serve.

Nutrition info per serving: calories 370, fat 11.7, fiber 4.2, carbs 8.9, protein 20

Pork Chops and Olives

Prep time: 10 minutes I **Cooking time:** 35 minutes I
Servings: 4

Ingredients:

- 4 pork chops
- 2 tablespoons olive oil
- 1 cup kalamata olives, pitted and halved
- 1 teaspoon allspice, ground
- ¼ cup coconut milk
- 1 yellow onion, chopped
- 1 tablespoon chives, chopped

Directions:

1. Heat up a pan with the oil over medium heat, add the onion and the meat and brown for 4 minutes on each side.
2. Add the rest of the ingredients, toss gently, introduce in the oven and bake at 390 degrees F for 25 minutes more.
3. Divide everything between plates and serve.

Nutrition info per serving: calories 290, fat 10, fiber 4.4, carbs 7.8, protein 22

Italian Lamb Chops

Prep time: 10 minutes I **Cooking time:** 30 minutes I
Servings: 4

Ingredients:

- 4 lamb chops
- 1 tablespoon oregano, chopped
- 1 tablespoon olive oil
- 1 yellow onion, chopped
- 2 tablespoons parmesan, grated
- 1/3 cup veggie stock
- Black pepper to the taste
- 1 teaspoon Italian seasoning

Directions:

1. Heat up a pan with the oil over medium-high heat, add the lamb chops and the onion and brown for 4 minutes on each side.
2. Add the rest of the ingredients except the cheese and toss.
3. Sprinkle the cheese on top, introduce the pan in the oven and bake at 350 degrees F for 20 minutes.
4. Divide everything between plates and serve.

Nutrition info per serving: calories 280, fat 17, fiber 5.5, carbs 11.2, protein 14

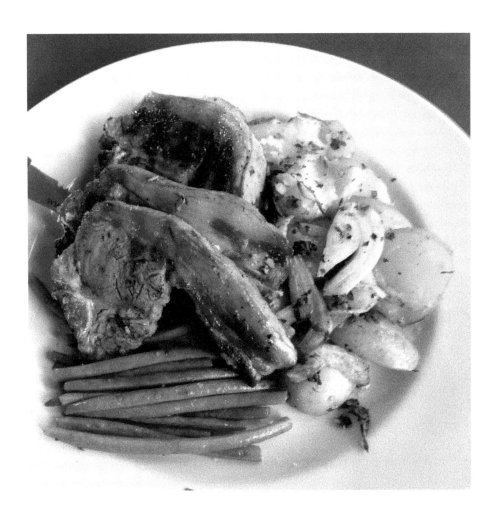

Pork and Lemon Rice

Prep time: 10 minutes I **Cooking time:** 35 minutes I
Servings: 4

Ingredients:

- 1 tablespoon olive oil
- 1 pound pork stew meat, cubed
- 1 tablespoon oregano, chopped
- 1 cup brown rice
- 2 cups chicken stock
- Black pepper to the taste
- 2 garlic cloves, minced
- Juice of ½ lemon
- 1 tablespoon cilantro, chopped

Directions:

1. Heat up a pot with the oil over medium heat, add the meat and the garlic and brown for 5 minutes.
2. Add the rice, the stock and the other ingredients, bring to a simmer and cook over medium heat for 30 minutes.
3. Divide everything between plates and serve.

Nutrition info per serving: calories 330, fat 13, fiber 5.2, carbs 13.4, protein 22.2

Pork Meatballs and Sauce

Prep time: 10 minutes I **Cooking time:** 30 minutes I
Servings: 4

Ingredients:

- 3 tablespoons almond flour
- 2 tablespoons avocado oil
- 2 egg, whisked
- Black pepper to the taste
- 2 pounds pork, ground
- 1 tablespoon cilantro, chopped
- 10 ounces tomato sauce

Directions:

1. In a bowl, combine the pork with the flour and the other ingredients except the sauce and the oil, stir well and shape medium meatballs out of this mix.
2. Heat up a pan with the oil over medium heat, add the meatballs and brown for 3 minutes on each   side. Add the sauce, toss gently, bring to a simmer and cook over medium heat for 20 minutes more.
3. Divide everything into bowls and serve.

Nutrition info per serving: calories 332, fat 18, fiber 4, carbs 14.3, protein 25

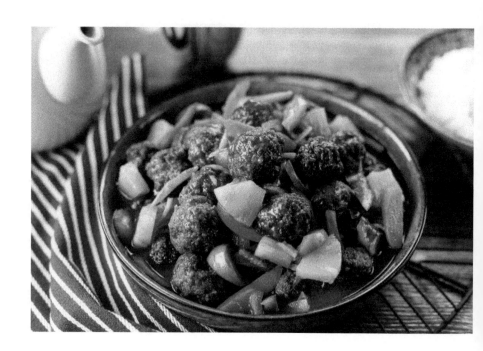

Pork and Endives

Prep time: 10 minutes I **Cooking time:** 35 minutes I **Servings:** 4

Ingredients:

- 1 pound pork stew meat, cubed
- 2 endives, trimmed and shredded
- 1 cup beef stock
- 1 teaspoon chili powder
- A pinch of black pepper
- 1 red onion, chopped
- 1 tablespoon olive oil

Directions:

1. Heat up a pan with the oil over medium heat, add the onion and the endives, toss and cook for 5 minutes.
2. Add the meat, toss and cook for 5 minutes more.
3. Add the rest of the ingredients, bring to a simmer and cook over medium heat for 25 minutes more.
4. Divide everything between plates and serve.

Nutrition info per serving: calories 330, fat 12.6, fiber 4.2, carbs 10, protein 22

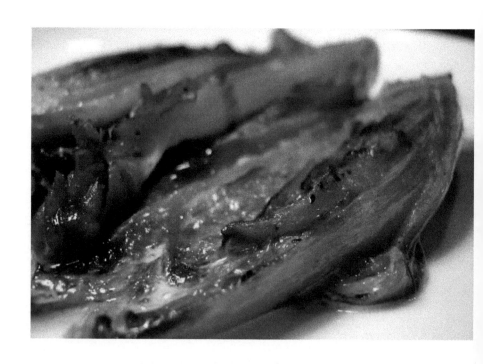

Pork and Radish Mix

Prep time: 10 minutes I **Cooking time:** 35 minutes I
Servings: 4

Ingredients:

- 1 cup radishes, cubed
- 1 pound pork stew meat, cubed
- 1 tablespoon olive oil
- 1 red onion, chopped
- 1 cup tomatoes, crushed
- 1 tablespoon chives, chopped
- 2 garlic cloves, minced
- Black pepper to the taste
- 1 teaspoon balsamic vinegar

Directions:

1. Heat up a pan with the oil over medium heat, add the onion and the garlic, stir and cook for 5 minutes.
2. Add the meat and brown for 5 minutes more.
3. Add the radishes and the other ingredients, bring to a simmer and cook over medium heat for 25 minutes more.
4. Divide everything into bowls and serve.

Nutrition info per serving: calories 274, fat 14, fiber 3.5, carbs 14.8, protein 24.1

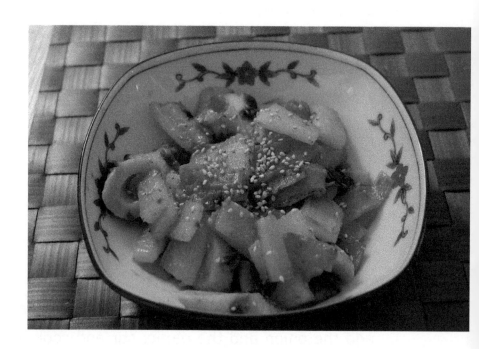

Mint Meatballs

Prep time: 10 minutes I **Cooking time:** 25 minutes I
Servings: 4

Ingredients:

- 1 pound pork stew meat, ground
- 1 yellow onion, chopped
- 1 egg, whisked
- 1 tablespoon mint, chopped
- Black pepper to the taste
- 2 garlic cloves, minced
- 2 tablespoons olive oil
- 1 cup cherry tomatoes, halved
- 1 cup baby spinach
- ½ cup veggie stock

Directions:

1. In a bowl, combine the meat with the onion and the other ingredients except the oil, cherry tomatoes and the spinach, stir well and shape medium meatballs out of this mix.
2. Heat up a pan with the olive oil over medium-high heat, add the meatballs and cook them for 5 minutes on each side.

3. Add the spinach, tomatoes and the stock, toss, simmer everything for 15 minutes.
4. Divide everything into bowls and serve.

Nutrition info per serving: calories 320, fat 13.4, fiber 6, carbs 15.8, protein 12

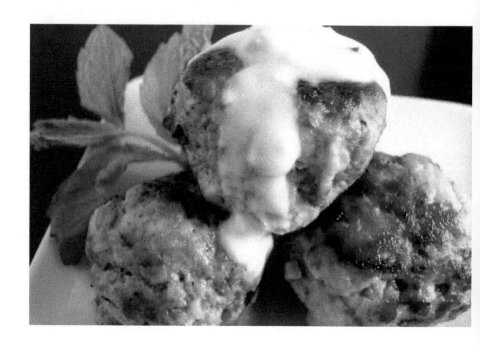

Meatballs and Sauce

Prep time: 10 minutes I **Cooking time:** 20 minutes I
Servings: 4

Ingredients:
- 2 pounds pork, ground
- Black pepper to the taste
- ¾ cup almond flour
- 2 eggs, whisked
- 1 tablespoon parsley, chopped
- 2 red onions, chopped
- 2 tablespoons olive oil
- ½ cup coconut cream
- Black pepper to the taste

Directions:
1. In a bowl, mix the pork with the almond flour and the other ingredients except the onions, oil and the cream, stir well and shape medium meatballs out of this mix.
2. Heat up a pan with the oil over medium heat, add the onions, stir and sauté for 5 minutes.
3. Add the meatballs, and cook for 5 minutes more.

4. Add coconut cream, bring to a simmer, cook everything for 10 minutes more, divide into bowls and serve.

Nutrition info per serving: calories 435, fat 23, fiber 14, carbs 33.2, protein 12.65

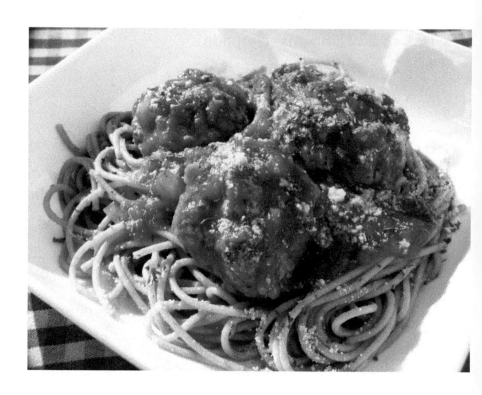

Pork and Lentils

Prep time: 10 minutes I **Cooking time:** 25 minutes I
Servings: 4

Ingredients:

- 1 pound pork stew meat, cubed
- ½ cup tomato sauce
- 1 yellow onion, chopped
- 2 tablespoons olive oil
- 1 cup lentils, cooked
- 1 teaspoon curry powder
- 1 teaspoon turmeric powder
- Black pepper to the taste

Directions:

1. Heat up a pan with the oil over medium-high heat, add the onion and the meat and brown for 5 minutes.
2. Add the sauce and the other ingredients, toss, cook over medium heat for 20 minutes, divide everything into bowls and serve.

Nutrition info per serving: calories 367, fat 23, fiber 6.9, carbs 22.1, protein 22

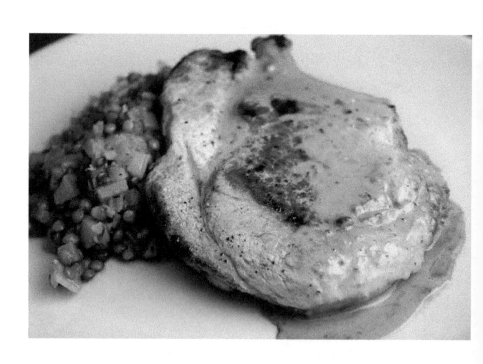

Lamb Pan

Prep time: 10 minutes I **Cooking time:** 25 minutes I
Servings: 4

Ingredients:

- 1 pound lamb meat, ground
- 1 tablespoon avocado oil
- 1 red bell pepper, cut into strips
- 1 red onion, sliced
- 2 tomatoes, cubed
- 1 carrot, cubed
- 2 fennel bulbs, sliced
- Black pepper to the taste
- 2 tablespoons balsamic vinegar
- 1 tablespoon cilantro, chopped

Directions:

1. Heat up a pan with the oil over medium-high heat, add the onion and the meat and brown for 5 minutes.
2. Add the bell pepper and the other ingredients, toss, cook over medium heat for 20 minutes more, divide into bowls and serve right away.

Nutrition info per serving: calories 367, fat 14.3, fiber 4.3, carbs 15.8, protein 16

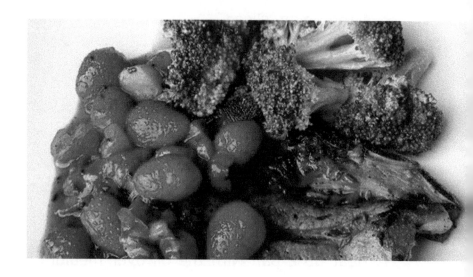

Coconut Pork with Beets

Prep time: 10 minutes I **Cooking time:** 30 minutes I
Servings: 4

Ingredients:
- 1 pound pork meat, cubed
- 2 small beets, peeled and cubed
- 2 tablespoons olive oil
- 1 yellow onion, chopped
- 2 garlic cloves, minced
- Salt and black pepper to the taste
- ½ cup coconut cream.

Directions:
1. Heat up a pan with the oil over medium-high heat, add the onion and the garlic, stir and cook for 5 minutes.
2. Add the meat and brown for 5 minutes more.
3. Add the rest of the ingredients, bring to a simmer and cook over medium heat for 20 minutes.
4. Divide the mix between plates and serve.

Nutrition info per serving: calories 311, fat 14.3, fiber 4.5, carbs 15.2, protein 17

Lamb and Tomato Cabbage Mix

Prep time: 10 minutes I **Cooking time:** 35 minutes I **Servings:** 4

Ingredients:

- 2 tablespoons avocado oil
- 1 pound lamb stew meat, roughly cubed
- 1 green cabbage head, shredded
- 1 cup tomatoes, chopped
- 1 yellow onion, chopped
- 1 teaspoon thyme, dried
- Black pepper to the taste
- 2 garlic cloves, minced

Directions:

1. Heat up a pan with the oil over medium-high heat, add the onion and garlic and sauté for 5 minutes.
2. Add the meat and brown for another 5 minutes.
3. Add the rest of the ingredients, toss, bring to a simmer and cook over medium heat for 25 minutes more.
4. Divide everything between plates and serve.

Nutrition info per serving: calories 325, fat 11, fiber 6.1, carbs 11.7, protein 16

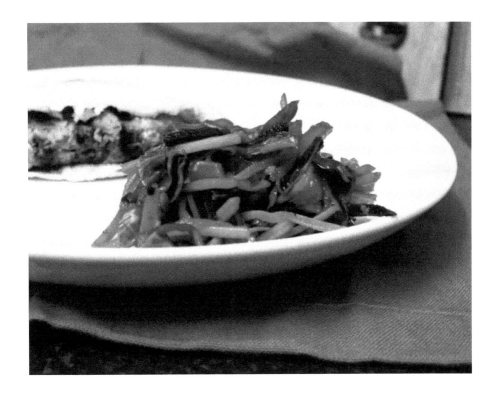

Lamb with Okra

Prep time: 10 minutes I **Cooking time:** 30 minutes I
Servings: 4

Ingredients:

- 1 pound lamb stew meat, roughly cubed
- 1 yellow onion, chopped
- 2 garlic cloves, minced
- 2 tablespoons avocado oil
- 1 cup okra, chopped
- 1 cup corn
- 1 cup veggie stock
- 1 tablespoon parsley, chopped

Directions:

1. Heat up a pan with the oil over medium-high heat, add the onion and the garlic, stir and sauté for 5 minutes.
2. Add the meat, toss and cook for 5 minutes more.
3. Add the rest of the ingredients, toss, bring to a simmer and cook over medium heat for 20 minutes.
4. Divide everything into bowls and serve.

Nutrition info per serving: calories 314, fat 12, fiber 4.4, carbs 13.3, protein 17

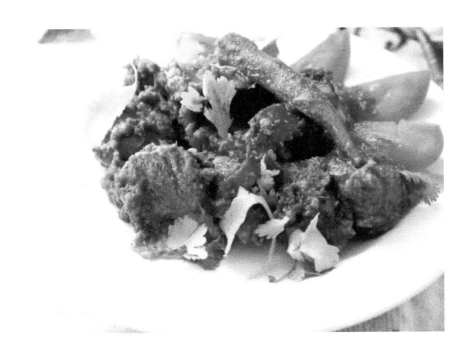

Mustard Pork

Prep time: 10 minutes I **Cooking time:** 8 hours I
Servings: 4

Ingredients:

- 2 pounds pork roast, sliced
- 2 tablespoons olive oil
- Black pepper to the taste
- 1 tablespoon tarragon, chopped
- 2 shallots, chopped
- 1 cup veggie stock
- 1 tablespoon thyme, chopped
- 1 tablespoon mustard

Directions:

1. In a slow cooker, combine the roast with the black pepper and the other ingredients, put the lid on and cook on Low for 8 hours.
2. Divide the pork roast between plates, drizzle the mustard sauce all over and serve.

Nutrition info per serving: calories 305, fat 14.5, fiber 5.4, carbs 15.7, protein 18

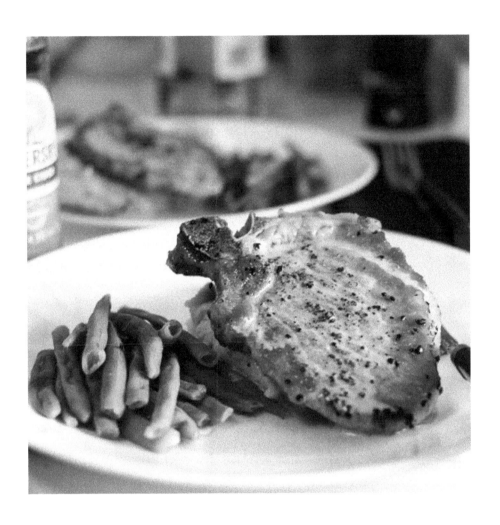

Pork with Capers

Prep time: 10 minutes I **Cooking time:** 35 minutes I
Servings: 4

Ingredients:

- 2 tablespoons olive oil
- 1 cup veggie stock
- 2 tablespoons capers, drained
- 1 pound pork chops
- 1 cup bean sprouts
- 1 yellow onion, cut into wedges
- Black pepper to the taste

Directions:

1. Heat up a pan with the oil over medium-high heat, add the onion and the meat and brown for 5 minutes.
2. Add the rest of the ingredients, introduce the pan in the oven and bake at 390 degrees F for 30 minutes.
3. Divide everything between plates and serve.

Nutrition info per serving: calories 324, fat 12.5, fiber 6.5, carbs 22.2, protein 15.6

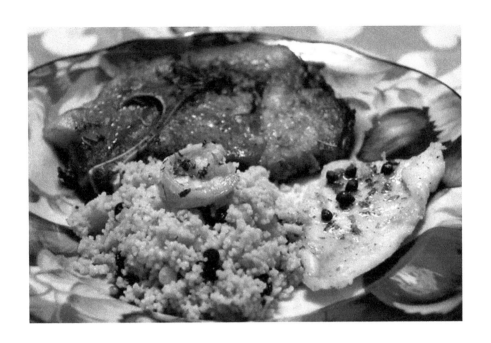

Pork with Spring Onions and Sprouts

Prep time: 10 minutes I **Cooking time:** 35 minutes I
Servings: 4

Ingredients:

- 2 pounds pork stew meat, cubed
- ¼ cup tomato sauce
- Black pepper to the taste
- ½ pound Brussels sprouts, halved
- 1 tablespoon olive oil
- 2 spring onions, chopped
- 1 tablespoon cilantro, chopped

Directions:

1. Heat up a pan with the oil over medium-high heat, add the onions and the sprouts and brown for 5 minutes.
2. Add the meat and the other ingredients, bring to a simmer and cook over medium heat for 30 minutes more.
3. Divide everything between plates and serve.

Nutrition info per serving: calories 541, fat 25.6, fiber 2.6, carbs 6.5, protein 68.7

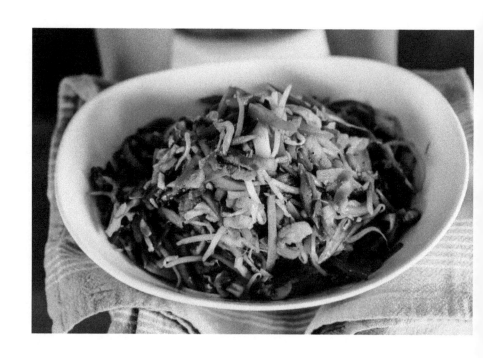

Pork and Hot Green Beans Mix

Prep time: 10 minutes I **Cooking time:** 20 minutes I
Servings: 4

Ingredients:

- 1 yellow onion, chopped
- 2 pounds pork meat, cut into strips
- ½ pound green beans, trimmed and halved
- 1 red bell pepper, chopped
- Black pepper to the taste
- 1 tablespoon olive oil
- ¼ cup red hot chili pepper, chopped
- 1 cup veggie stock

Directions:

1. Heat up a pan with the oil over medium-high heat, add the onion and sauté for 5 minutes.
2. Add the meat and brown for 5 minutes more.
3. Add the rest of the ingredients, toss, cook for 10 minutes over medium heat, divide between plates and serve.

Nutrition info per serving: calories 347, fat 24.8, fiber 3.3, carbs 18.1, protein 15.2

Lamb with Quinoa

Prep time: 10 minutes I **Cooking time:** 30 minutes I
Servings: 4

Ingredients:

- 1 cup quinoa
- 2 cups chicken stock
- 1 tablespoon olive oil
- 1 cup coconut cream
- 2 pounds lamb stew meat, cubed
- 2 shallots, chopped
- 2 garlic cloves, minced
- Black pepper to the taste
- A pinch of red pepper flakes, crushed

Directions:

1. Heat up a pot with the oil over medium-high heat, add the shallots and the garlic, stir and sauté for 5 minutes.
2. Add the meat and brown for 5 minutes more.
3. Add the rest of the ingredients, stir, bring to a simmer, reduce heat to medium and cook for 20 minutes.
4. Divide the mix bowls and serve.

Nutrition info per serving: calories 755, fat 37, fiber 4.4, carbs 32, protein 71.8

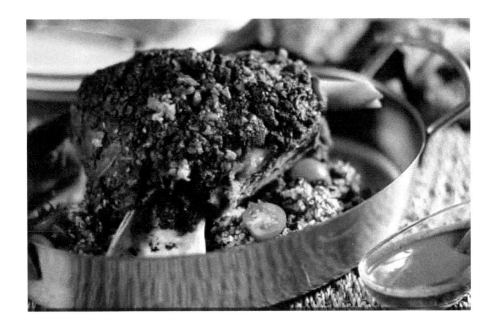

Lamb and Bok Choy

Prep time: 10 minutes I **Cooking time:** 30 minutes I
Servings: 4

Ingredients:

- 1 cup chicken stock
- 1 cup bok choy, torn
- 1 pound lamb stew meat, roughly cubed
- 2 tablespoons avocado oil
- 1 yellow onion, chopped
- 1 carrot, chopped
- Black pepper to the taste

Directions:

1. Heat up a pan with the oil over medium-high heat, add the onion and the carrot and sauté for 5 minutes.
2. Add the meat and brown for 5 minutes more.
3. Add the rest of the ingredients, bring to a simmer and cook over medium heat for 20 minutes.
4. Divide everything between plates and serve.

Nutrition info per serving: calories 360, fat 14.5, fiber 5, carbs 22.4, protein 16

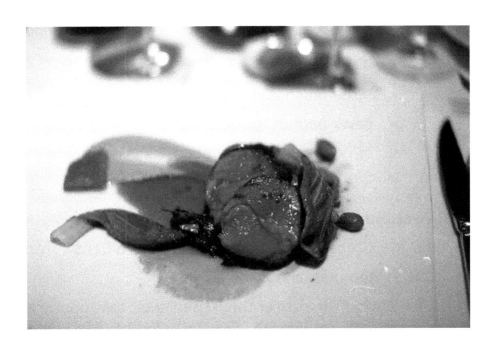

Coconut Pork with Okra and Olives

Prep time: 10 minutes I **Cooking time:** 35 minutes I
Servings: 4

Ingredients:

- ½ cup veggie stock
- 1 cup okra, trimmed
- 1 cup black olives, pitted and halved
- 2 tablespoons olive oil
- 4 pork chops
- 1 red onion, cut into wedges
- Black pepper to the taste
- ½ tablespoon red pepper flakes
- 3 tablespoons coconut aminos

Directions:

1. Grease a roasting pan with the oil and arrange the pork chops inside.
2. Add the rest of the ingredients, toss gently and bake at 390 degrees F for 35 minutes.
3. Divide everything between plates and serve.

Nutrition info per serving: calories 310, fat 14.6, fiber 6, carbs 20.4, protein 16

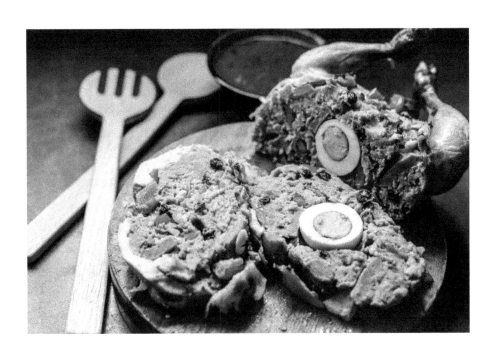

Pork and Barley

Prep time: 10 minutes I **Cooking time:** 35 minutes I
Servings: 4

Ingredients:

- 1 cup barley
- 2 cups chicken stock
- 1 pound pork stew meat, cubed
- 1 red onion, sliced
- 1 tablespoon olive oil
- Black pepper to the taste
- 1 teaspoon fenugreek powder
- 1 tablespoon chives, chopped
- 1 tablespoon capers, drained

Directions:

1. Heat up a pan with the oil over medium-high heat, add the onion and the meat and brown for 5 minutes.
2. Add the barley and the other ingredients, toss, bring to a simmer cook over medium heat for 30 minutes.
3. Divide everything into bowls and serve.

Nutrition info per serving: calories 447, fat 15.6, fiber 8.6, carbs 36.5, protein 39.8

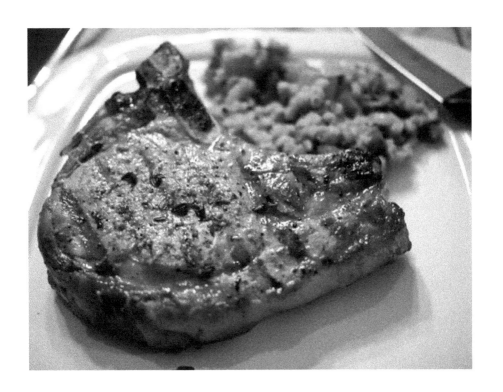

Pork and Green Onions

Prep time: 10 minutes I **Cooking time:** 40 minutes I
Servings: 5

Ingredients:

- 1 pound pork meat, cubed
- 1 tablespoon avocado oil
- 1 yellow onion, chopped
- 1 bunch green onion, chopped
- 4 garlic cloves, minced
- 1 cup tomato sauce
- Black pepper to the taste

Directions:

1. Heat up a pan with the oil over medium-high heat, add the onion and green onions, stir and cook for 5 minutes.
2. Add the meat, stir and cook for 5 minutes more.
3. Add the rest of the ingredients, toss and cook over medium heat for 30 minutes more.
4. Divide everything into bowls and serve.

Nutrition info per serving: calories 206, fat 8.6, fiber 1.8, carbs 7.2, protein 23.4

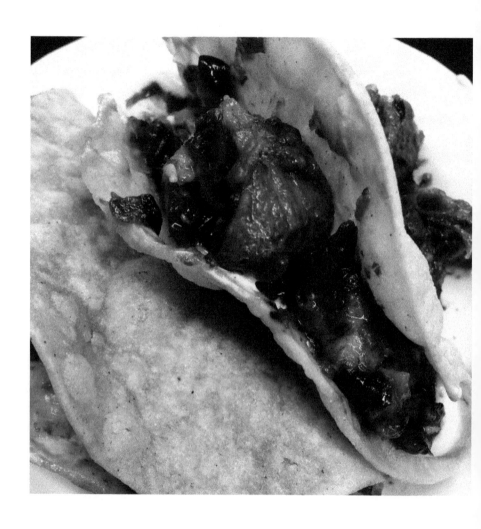

Pork and Black Beans

Prep time: 5 minutes I **Cooking time:** 40 minutes I
Servings: 8

Ingredients:

- 2 tablespoons olive oil
- 1 cup black beans, cooked
- 1 yellow onion, chopped
- 1 cup tomatoes , chopped
- 2 pounds pork stew meat, cubed
- 2 garlic cloves, minced
- Black pepper to the taste
- ½ teaspoon nutmeg, ground

Directions:

1. Heat up a pan with the oil over medium heat, add the onion and the garlic and sauté for 5 minutes.
2. Add the meat, toss and cook for 5 minutes more.
3. Add the rest of the ingredients, toss, bring to a simmer and cook over medium heat for 30 minutes.
4. Divide the mix into bowls and serve.

Nutrition info per serving: calories 365, fat 14.9, fiber 4.3, carbs 17.6, protein 38.8

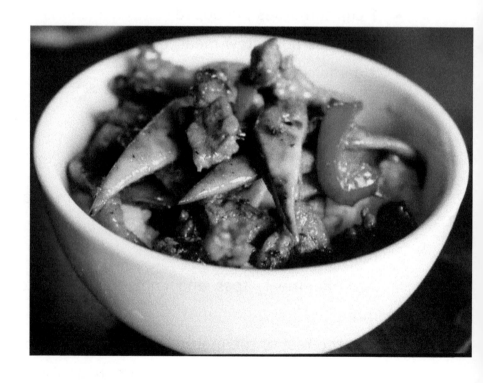

Dill Chicken

Prep time: 10 minutes I **Cooking time:** 45 minutes I

Servings: 4

Ingredients:

- 2 tablespoons olive oil
- 1 yellow onion, chopped
- 2 pounds chicken thighs, skinless, boneless
- 4 garlic cloves, minced
- ½ cup chicken stock
- 1 teaspoon turmeric powder
- 1 leek, sliced
- A pinch of salt and black pepper
- 3 tablespoons dill, chopped
- 2 tablespoons lemon juice

Directions:

1. Heat up a pan with the oil over medium heat, add the onion, garlic and leek and sauté for 5 minutes.
2. Add the meat and brown for 5 minutes more.
3. Add the rest of the ingredients, toss, introduce the pan in the oven and bake at 380 degrees F for 35 minutes.
4. Divide everything between plates and serve.

Nutrition info per serving: calories 531, fat 24.2, fiber 1.5, carbs 8.6, protein 67.1

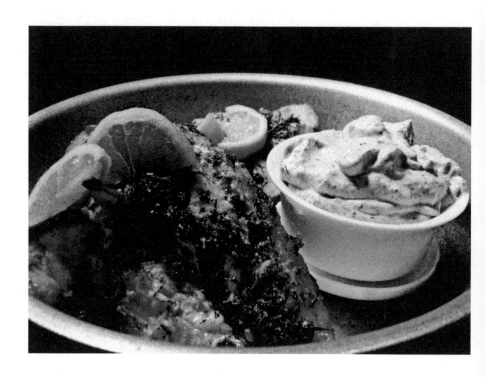

Turkey and Onions Mix

Prep time: 5 minutes I **Cooking time:** 8 hours I
Servings: 4

Ingredients:

- 2 pounds turkey breast, skinless, boneless and sliced
- 1 cup blackberries
- 2 yellow onions, sliced
- 2 tablespoons olive oil
- ½ cup chicken stock
- ½ teaspoon chili powder
- 1 teaspoon sweet paprika
- A pinch of salt and black pepper
- 4 garlic cloves, minced
- 1 tablespoon parsley, chopped

Directions:

1. In a slow cooker, combine the turkey with the blackberries and the other ingredients, toss gently, put the lid on and cook on Low for 8 hours.
2. Divide the mix between plates and serve.

Nutrition info per serving: calories 331, fat 11.2, fiber 4, carbs 17.2, protein 39.9

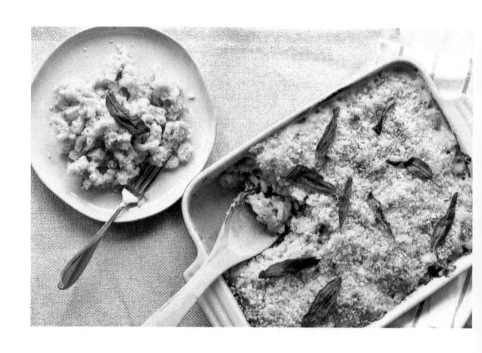

Turkey with Almonds and Leeks

Prep time: 5 minutes I **Cooking time:** 30 minutes I
Servings: 4

Ingredients:

- 2 pounds turkey breast, skinless, boneless and cubed
- 2 leeks, sliced
- 1 tablespoon olive oil
- 2 teaspoons coriander, chopped
- A pinch of salt and black pepper
- 2 garlic clove, minced
- 2 tablespoons balsamic vinegar
- 2 tablespoons almonds, chopped
- 1 tablespoon cilantro, chopped

Directions:

1. Heat up a pan with the oil over medium-high heat, add the leeks and the garlic and sauté for 5 minutes.
2. Add the turkey and brown for 5 minutes more.
3. Add the rest of the ingredients, toss, cook over medium heat for 20 minutes, divide between plates and serve.

Nutrition info per serving: calories 320, fat 9, fiber 3, carbs 18, protein 40.6

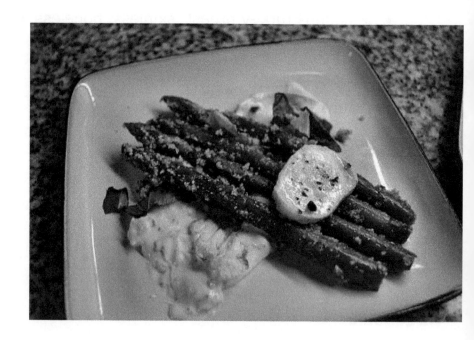

Chicken and Zucchini

Prep time: 5 minutes I **Cooking time:** 35 minutes I
Servings: 4

Ingredients:

- 1 pound chicken breast, skinless, boneless and ground
- 1 yellow onion, chopped
- 2 tablespoons olive oil
- 2 zucchinis, sliced
- 2 garlic cloves, minced
- 2 cups tomatoes, cubed
- ½ cup tomato paste
- 1 cup chicken stock
- 1 teaspoon chili powder
- 1 teaspoon cumin, ground
- 1 teaspoon rosemary, dried
- A pinch of salt and black pepper
- 1 tablespoon cilantro, chopped

Directions:

1. Heat up a pot with the oil over medium-high heat, add the onion and the garlic and sauté for 5 minutes.
2. Add the meat and brown for 5 minutes more.

3. Add the zucchinis and the other ingredients, toss, bring to a simmer and cook over medium heat for 25 minutes.
4. Divide the chili into bowls and serve.

Nutrition info per serving: calories 269, fat 10.8, fiber 4.6, carbs 17, protein 28.2

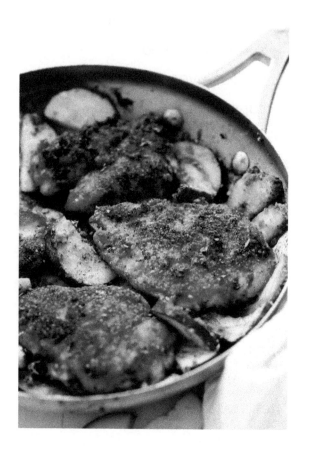

Creamy Turkey

Prep time: 10 minutes I **Cooking time:** 30 minutes I
Servings: 4

Ingredients:

- 1 pound turkey breast, skinless, boneless and cubed
- 1 yellow onion, chopped
- 2 tablespoons avocado oil
- 1 teaspoon chili powder
- A pinch of salt and black pepper
- 1 cup coconut cream
- 1 tablespoon lime zest, grated
- 2 tablespoons lime juice
- 3 garlic cloves, minced
- 2 green chilies, chopped

Directions:

1. Heat up a pan with the oil over medium-high heat, add onion, garlic, chilies and chili powder and sauté for 5 minutes.
2. Add the meat and cook it for 5 minutes more.
3. Add the remaining ingredients, toss, bring to a simmer and cook over medium heat for 20 minutes more.

4. Divide everything between plates and serve.

Nutrition info per serving: calories 283, fat 17.2, fiber 3.3, carbs 12.6, protein 21.4

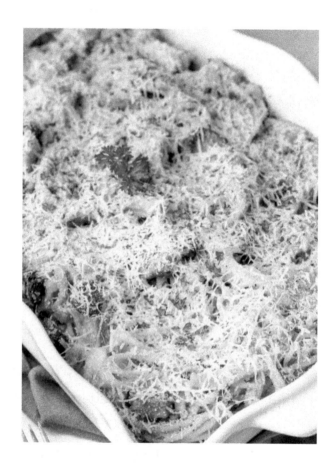

Chicken and Squash

Prep time: 10 minutes I **Cooking time:** 40 minutes I
Servings: 4

Ingredients:

- 2 pounds chicken breast, skinless, boneless and sliced
- 1 yellow onion, chopped
- 2 tablespoons olive oil
- 2 garlic cloves, minced
- 1 teaspoon turmeric powder
- ½ teaspoon cumin, ground
- ½ teaspoon fennel seeds, crushed
- 14 ounces tomatoes, chopped
- 1 teaspoon oregano, dried
- 1 teaspoon chili powder
- A pinch of salt and black pepper
- 2 cups butternut squash, peeled and cubed
- 2 tablespoons cilantro, chopped

Directions:

1. Heat up a pot with the oil over medium-high heat, add the onion and the garlic and sauté for 5 minutes.
2. Add the meat and brown it for 5 minutes more.

3. Add the cumin, turmeric, the squash and the other ingredients, toss, bring to a simmer and cook over medium heat for 30 minutes more.
4. Divide the whole mix between plates and serve.

Nutrition info per serving: calories 261, fat 4, fiber 8, carbs 15, protein 7

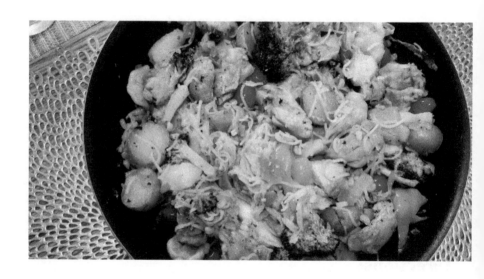

Chicken with Basil Beans

Prep time: 10 minutes I **Cooking time:** 40 minutes I
Servings: 4

Ingredients:

- 2 pounds chicken breasts, skinless, boneless and cubed
- 1 cup black beans, cooked
- 1 cup red kidney beans, cooked
- 1 yellow onion, chopped
- 2 tablespoons avocado oil
- A pinch of salt and black pepper
- 1 teaspoon smoked paprika
- 1 teaspoon basil, dried
- 1 cup chicken stock
- 1 cup tomatoes, crushed
- 1 tablespoon parsley, chopped

Directions:

1. Heat up a pan with the oil over medium-high heat, add the onion and sauté for 5 minutes.
2. Add the meat and brown it for 5 minutes more.
3. Add the beans and the other ingredients, toss, reduce heat to medium and cook everything for 30 minutes more.

4. Divide the mix between plates and serve.

Nutrition info per serving: calories 312, fat 7, fiber 7, carbs 15, protein 15

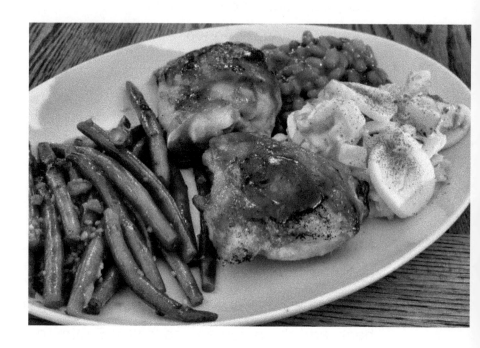

Turkey and Rice

Prep time: 10 minutes I **Cooking time:** 40 minutes I
Servings: 4

Ingredients:

- 2 pounds turkey breast, skinless, boneless and cubed
- 1 yellow onion, chopped
- 2 tablespoons olive oil
- 3 garlic cloves, minced
- A pinch of salt and black pepper
- 1 cup black rice
- 3 cups chicken stock
- 1 tablespoon basil, chopped
- ½ teaspoon cumin, ground
- 1 teaspoon chili powder
- 1 teaspoon rosemary, dried
- 1 tablespoon thyme, chopped

Directions:

1. Heat up a pot with the oil over medium-high heat, add the onion and the garlic and sauté for 5 minutes.
2. Add the meat and brown for 5 minutes more.

3. Add the rice, stock and the other ingredients, toss, bring to a simmer and cook over medium heat for 30 minutes.
4. Divide the mix between plates and serve right away.

Nutrition info per serving: calories 251, fat 4, fiber 7, carbs 13, protein 5

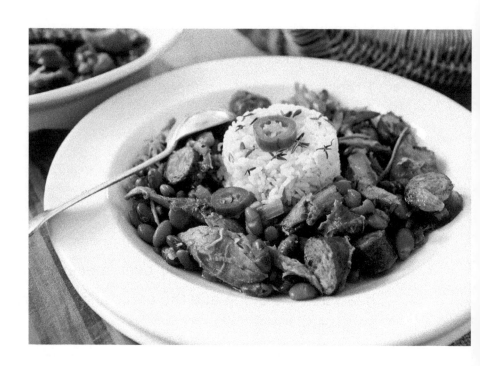

Chicken with Mint Mushrooms Mix

Prep time: 5 minutes I **Cooking time:** 45 minutes I
Servings: 4

Ingredients:

- 1 yellow onion, chopped
- 2 tablespoons avocado oil
- 2 pounds chicken breast, skinless, boneless and sliced
- 2 cups white mushrooms, sliced
- A pinch of salt and black pepper
- ¼ cup mint, chopped
- 2 garlic cloves, minced
- 1 teaspoon coriander, ground
- ½ teaspoon cayenne pepper
- 1 tablespoon sweet paprika
- 1 tablespoon lemon juice

Directions:

1. Heat up a pan with the oil over medium-high heat, add the onion and the garlic and sauté for 5 minutes.
2. Add the mushrooms and cook them for 5 minutes more.

3. Add the chicken and sauté for another 5 minutes.

4. Add the rest of the ingredients, put the pan in the oven and bake at 380 degrees F for 30 minutes.

5. Divide everything between plates and serve.

Nutrition info per serving: calories 251, fat 4, fiber 6, carbs 15, protein 7

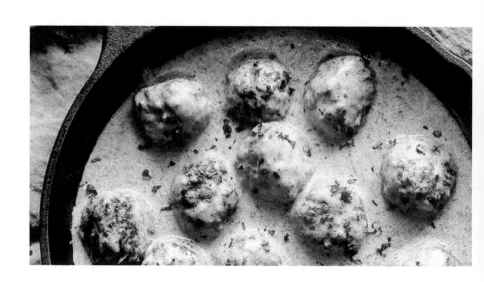

Chicken and Garlic Peas

Prep time: 10 minutes I **Cooking time:** 40 minutes I
Servings: 4

Ingredients:

- 2 pounds chicken breast, skinless, boneless and sliced
- 4 scallions, chopped
- 2 tablespoons olive oil
- 2 cups sugar snap peas
- 2 garlic cloves, minced
- 1 teaspoon cayenne pepper
- ½ teaspoon hot paprika
- 2 tablespoons balsamic vinegar
- 1 tablespoon sesame seeds, toasted
- 1 tablespoon cilantro, chopped

Directions:

1. Heat up a pan with the olive oil over medium-high heat, add the scallions and the garlic and sauté for 5 minutes.
2. Add the meat and brown for 5 minutes more.
3. Add the snap peas and the rest of the ingredients, toss, cook over medium heat for

30 minutes more, divide between plates and serve.

Nutrition info per serving: calories 261, fat 2, fiber 6, carbs 15, protein 6

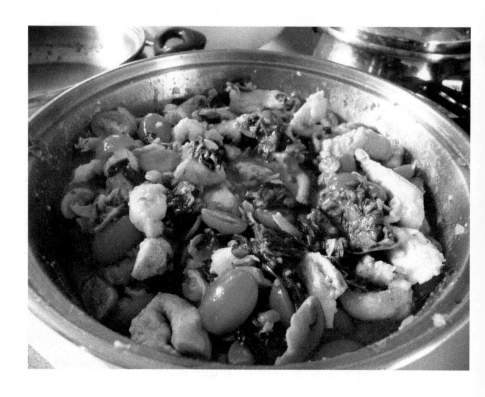

Turkey with Parsley Chickpeas

Prep time: 10 minutes I **Cooking time:** 35 minutes I
Servings: 4

Ingredients:
- 1 sweet onion, chopped
- 4 garlic cloves, minced
- 1 pound turkey breast, skinless, boneless and cubed
- 2 tablespoons olive oil
- 1 cup chickpeas, cooked
- 1 cup chicken stock
- 2 tablespoons lemon juice
- A pinch of salt and black pepper
- 1 tablespoon parsley, chopped

Directions:
1. Heat up a pan with the oil over medium-high heat, add the onion, garlic and the meat and brown for 10 minutes.
2. Add the rest of the ingredients, toss, cook over medium heat for 25 minutes more, divide between plates and serve.

Nutrition info per serving: calories 272, fat 5, fiber 6, carbs 15, protein 6

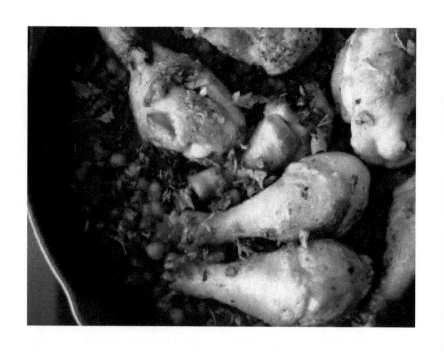

Turkey and Basil Cucumber Mix

Prep time: 5 minutes I **Cooking time:** 35 minutes I
Servings: 4

Ingredients:

- 2 pounds turkey breast, skinless, boneless and sliced
- 2 tablespoons olive oil
- 1 yellow onion, chopped
- 2 teaspoons Italian seasoning
- 1 teaspoon coriander, ground
- ½ teaspoon basil, dried
- A pinch of salt and black pepper
- 2 cucumbers, sliced
- 1 tablespoon cilantro, chopped

Directions:

1. Heat up a pan with the oil over medium-high heat, add the onion and sauté for 5 minutes.
2. Add the meat and brown for 5 minutes more.
3. Add the rest of the ingredients, toss, introduce in the oven and bake at 400 degrees F for 25 minutes more.
4. Divide the mix between plates and serve.

Nutrition info per serving: calories 277, fat 4, fiber 4, carbs 14, protein 8

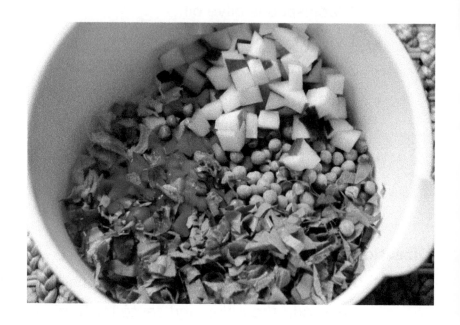

Chicken with Spinach

Prep time: 5 minutes I **Cooking time:** 35 minutes I
Servings: 4

Ingredients:

- 2 pounds chicken thighs, skinless, boneless and cubed
- 1 yellow onion, chopped
- 2 tablespoons olive oil
- A pinch of salt and black pepper
- 1 cup baby spinach
- 1 fennel bulb, sliced
- ½ teaspoon fennel seeds, crushed
- ½ teaspoon coriander, ground
- ½ cup chicken stock
- 1 tablespoon cilantro, chopped
- 1 tablespoon chives, chopped

Directions:

1. Heat up a pan with the oil over medium-high heat, add the onion and the fennel and sauté for 5 minutes.
2. Add the chicken and brown for 5 minutes more.

3. Add the fennel seeds and the other ingredients, toss, bring to a simmer and cook over medium heat for 25 minutes more.
4. Divide the mix between plates and serve.

Nutrition info per serving: calories 288, fat 4, fiber 6, carbs 12, protein 7

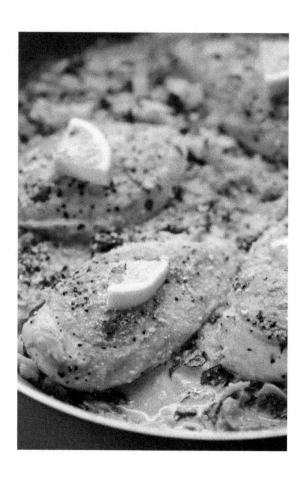

Chicken with Peppers

Prep time: 10 minutes I **Cooking time:** 40 minutes I
Servings: 4

Ingredients:

- 1 pound chicken breasts, skinless, boneless and sliced
- 1 red bell pepper, sliced
- 2 tablespoons olive oil
- 1 green bell pepper, sliced
- 1 yellow onion, chopped
- 1 cup black olives, pitted and halved
- 4 garlic cloves, minced
- 1 bay leaf
- 1 teaspoon black peppercorns
- A pinch of salt and black pepper
- 1 tablespoon balsamic vinegar

Directions:

1. In a roasting pan, combine the chicken with the bell peppers and the other ingredients, toss a bit, introduce in the oven and bake at 380 degrees F for 40 minutes.
2. Divide the mix between plates and serve.

Nutrition info per serving: calories 221, fat 4, fiber 5, carbs 14, protein 11

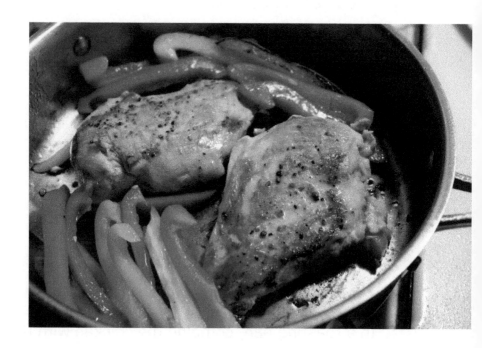

Turkey with Quinoa

Prep time: 10 minutes I **Cooking time:** 40 minutes I
Servings: 4

Ingredients:

- 1 pound turkey breast, skinless, boneless and sliced
- 1 cup quinoa
- 3 cups chicken stock
- ½ cup radish, sliced
- 2 tablespoons olive oil
- A pinch of salt and black pepper
- 4 scallions, chopped
- ¼ cup basil, torn

Directions:

1. Heat up a pan with the oil over medium-high heat, add the scallions and the meat and brown for 5 minutes.
2. Add the quinoa and the other ingredients, toss, bring to a simmer and cook over medium heat for 35 minutes.
3. Divide everything between plates and serve.

Nutrition info per serving: calories 213, fat 3, fiber 5, carbs 9, protein 6

Rosemary Lemon Chicken

Prep time: 10 minutes I **Cooking time:** 8 hours I
Servings: 4

Ingredients:

- 1 yellow onion, sliced
- 2 pounds chicken thighs, boneless and skinless
- 2 tablespoons olive oil
- A pinch of salt and black pepper
- 1 rosemary bunch, torn
- Juice of ½ lemon
- ½ cup tomatoes, cubed

Directions:

1. In your slow cooker, combine the chicken with the oil and the other ingredients, toss and cook on Low for 8 hours.
2. Divide the mix between plates and serve.

Nutrition info per serving: calories 300, fat 7, fiber 4, carbs 15, protein 20

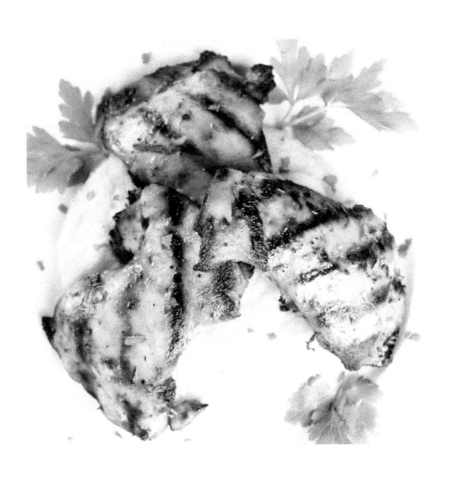

Chicken and Paprika Cherries Mix

Prep time: 5 minutes I **Cooking time:** 30 minutes I **Servings:** 4

Ingredients:

- 1 pound chicken breasts, skinless, boneless and sliced
- A pinch of salt and black pepper
- 2 tablespoons lemon juice
- 1 tablespoon lemon zest, grated
- 2 tablespoons olive oil
- 1 teaspoon sweet paprika
- 2 cups sweet cherries, pitted and chopped
- 1 tablespoon cilantro, chopped

Directions:

1. Heat up a pan with the oil over medium heat, add the chicken and brown for 5 minutes.
2. Add the rest of the ingredients, toss, cook over medium heat for 25 minutes more, divide between plates and serve.

Nutrition info per serving: calories 227, fat 3, fiber 6, carbs 15, protein 9

Duck and Chili Cauliflower

Prep time: 10 minutes I **Cooking time:** 35 minutes I
Servings: 4

Ingredients:

- 1 yellow onion, chopped
- 1 pound duck breast, boneless and skin scored
- 2 tablespoons olive oil
- 2 tablespoons parsley, chopped
- 4 garlic cloves, minced
- A pinch of salt and black pepper
- Juice of 1 lemon
- ½ pound cauliflower florets
- 1 teaspoon chili powder
- ½ teaspoon red pepper, crushed

Directions:

1. Heat up a pan with the oil over medium-high heat, add the onion and sauté for 5 minutes.
2. Add the duck, skin side down and cook for 5 minutes more.
3. Add the rest of the ingredients, toss, cook over medium heat for 25 minutes more, divide between plates and serve.

Nutrition info per serving: calories 278, fat 14, fiber 6, carbs 14, protein 27

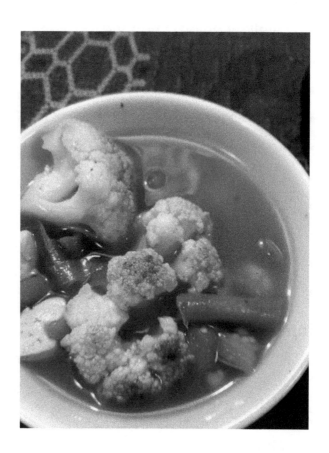

Chicken with Cilantro Peaches

Prep time: 10 minutes I **Cooking time:** 30 minutes I
Servings: 4

Ingredients:

- 1 yellow onion, chopped
- 2 tablespoons olive oil
- 1 pound chicken breast, skinless, boneless and sliced
- 1 cup peaches, peeled and cubed
- 3 tablespoons lime juice
- A pinch of salt and black pepper
- 1 tablespoon lime zest, grated
- 1 tablespoon cilantro, chopped

Directions:

1. Heat up a pan with the oil over medium-high heat, add the onion and sauté for 5 minutes.
2. Add the meat and brown for 5 minutes more.
3. Add the rest of the ingredients, toss, cook over medium heat for 20 minutes, divide between plates and serve.

Nutrition info per serving: calories 271, fat 4, fiber 8, carbs 16, protein 8

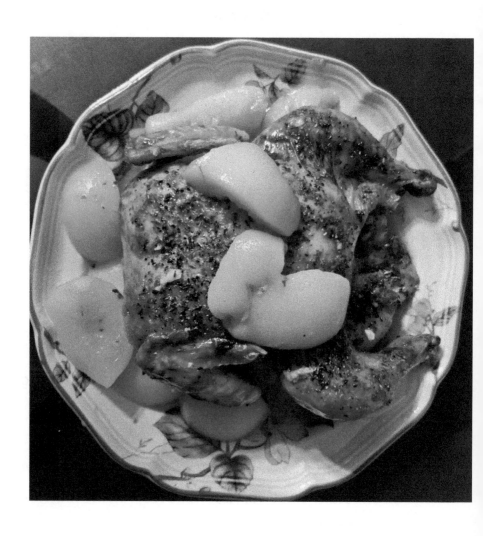

Chicken with Parsley Tomato Rice

Prep time: 10 minutes I **Cooking time:** 30 minutes I
Servings: 4

Ingredients:

- 1 yellow onion, chopped
- 2 tablespoons olive oil
- 1 pound chicken breast, skinless, boneless and cubed
- 1 tablespoon lemon zest, grated
- 2 tablespoons lemon juice
- 3 garlic cloves, minced
- 1 cup brown rice
- 2 cups chicken stock
- ½ cup grape tomatoes, halved
- 1 tablespoon parsley, chopped

Directions:

1. Heat up a pan with the oil over medium heat, add the onion and sauté for 5 minutes.
2. Add the meat and brown for 5 minutes.
3. Add the rest of the ingredients, toss, cook everything for 20 minutes more, divide between plates and serve.

Nutrition info per serving: calories 288, fat 6, fiber 5, carbs 14, protein 20

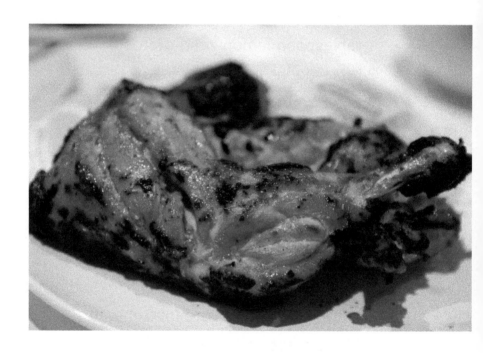

Turkey with Asparagus

Prep time: 10 minutes I **Cooking time:** 30 minutes I
Servings: 4

Ingredients:

- 1 pound turkey breast, skinless, boneless and sliced
- 2 tablespoons olive oil
- 4 scallions, chopped
- A pinch of salt and black pepper
- 1 cup chicken stock
- ¼ cup tomato sauce
- 1 bunch asparagus, sliced
- 2 teaspoons lemon juice
- 2 garlic cloves, minced
- 1 tablespoon coriander, chopped

Directions:

1. Heat up a pan with the oil over medium-high heat, add the scallions and the garlic and sauté for 5 minutes.
2. Add the meat and brown for 5 minutes more.
3. Add the rest of the ingredients, toss, cook over medium heat for 20 minutes more, divide between plates and serve.

Nutrition info per serving: calories 271, fat 6, fiber 7, carbs 8, protein 16

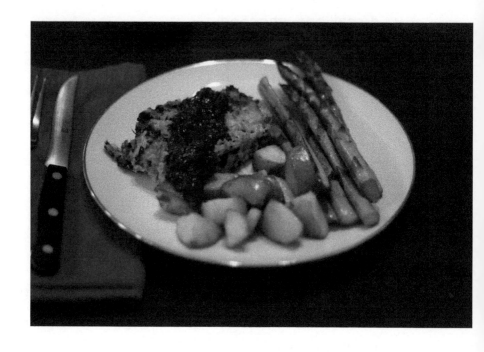